Emergency Preparation

What to Do When an Emergency Strikes Your Family

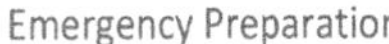

Table of Contents

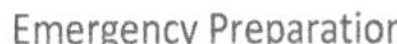

Why should one always be ready?

The possibility of being affected by a natural disaster is always present and can strike at any time and in any part of the world.Experiencing a disaster is a terrible experience in and of itself; having the additional disadvantage of being unprepared for such an incident will ultimately result in more unnecessary stress being added to a situation that is already unpleasant.

Being well-prepared for an unexpected event offers a number of distinct advantages.

If you are prepared for a circumstance, you will have a much easier time coping with the worry, stress, and anxiety that are normally triggered by it.You may guarantee that these sensations are kept to a minimum by ensuring that you are prepared and that you are familiar with the procedures that are carried out during these types of circumstances.

If a person is under a significant level of stress and worry, it is possible that they will be unable to react appropriately or efficiently when confronted with a problem. It is quite improbable that you will be able to adequately take care of yourself and your family if you are unable to think and behave in an appropriate manner. You will increase your chances of being able to respond in an appropriate manner to various kinds of emergency situations if you are prepared with the appropriate equipment and if you familiarize yourself with the characteristics, requirements, and procedures that apply during those kinds of emergency situations.

You have a better chance of successfully reducing the negative effects of a circumstance if you are well-prepared and are aware of the potential outcomes of various scenarios before they occur. For instance, if you educate yourself about the features of a cyclone, you will be better prepared to protect your belongings and find shelter in the event that you ever find yourself in a situation similar to this one. As a result, you will be able to successfully limit the amount of damage caused by the cyclone.

What should I do to get ready?

There are a variety of approaches you may take in order to effectively plan for an unexpected circumstance and guarantee that you are well prepared for the occurrence of the event. If you are able to maximize your degree of organization, you will ultimately be able to respond efficiently to an emergency scenario, which will, God willing, help in the effort to reduce the amount of damage caused by a disaster.

In order to be ready for any emergency, the first step is to educate yourself on the potential hazards that may arise in the region of the country or state in which you live. In the event of an emergency, it is important to be aware of the risk and warning signs as well as the procedures that are followed locally.

If you are aware with the different sorts of natural disasters that could take place in your region, then you will have sufficient knowledge with which to organize emergency procedures for the catastrophes that are relevant to you. You will also find that it is helpful in the process of putting together an emergency supply kit.

Before a catastrophe occurs, it is important to be aware of a few aspects that could prove to be helpful.

To get started, you should do some study on various natural disasters that could potentially affect the region in which you live. You may try searching for the information you need on the internet, where you might discover a substantial amount of it; alternatively, you could get in touch with the right weather bureau and inquire as to whether they could provide you the essential information. Discuss the matter with your fellow community members and close friends.

After you have gathered adequate information on any potential disasters, you can then begin establishing protocols for yourself and your family to adhere to in the event of one of those disasters. When it comes to making preparations for an emergency, you should keep the following in mind as some of the elements you ought to take into account:

1) Evacuation routes: Walk around your home or make a floor plan to locate potential exits that are suitable for a variety of emergencies. Aim to have two exits leading out of every separate room.

2) Where to congregate: In the event of a crisis, every member of the family may have to leave the house via a separate room. Determine a spot that is suitable for everyone to congregate in so that you can guarantee a safe evacuation.

3) Communication: If a disaster were to occur, the best possible time for it would be during a time when the entire family is together. However, since this is unlikely to occur, you should be ready for it and establish a means of communication or designate a meeting site. Talk about how you will communicate in a number of different settings when you meet.

4) Procedures Already in Place Be familiar with any and all emergency procedures that may be in place at the location where you work or where your children attend school. This can be helpful in organizing a means of contact or a specific meeting place for you.

5) Put together a disaster supplies kit. This will ensure that you are fully prepared in the event of a disaster and will prevent you from having to search around and obtain relevant items in the midst of a disaster, when you may not be thinking effectively due to the stress and anxiety that has resulted from the disaster. For additional information on how to make an emergency supplies kit as well as what goods you will require, please refer to chapter three.

6) Be aware of how to shut off the water or gas supply to your home in an emergency. This might come in handy in the case that there is an evacuation.

7) Designating some rooms as "shelter" areas We frequently hear that people need to take shelter when we hear about natural disasters. The phrase "taking shelter" can mean either taking shelter in one's own home or taking shelter outside of a specific location. It is always to one's advantage to plan ahead and designate specific areas of one's home as "safe" for use in a variety of emergency scenarios. In the event that you are forced to leave your house, it is a good idea to make preparations for alternative types of shelter (such as staying with a relative, checking into a hotel, etc.).

8) Insurance: If a calamity were to strike and cause damage to your home or its contents, you should make sure to get the appropriate insurance so that you would have a way to replace your belongings. You should compile an inventory of your belongings for the purpose of obtaining insurance; the most efficient ways to do so are by composing a list and either taking images or video of your valuables.
Obtaining insurance coverage for one's health and one's life could also be advantageous

9) Safekeeping of vital records Make sure that all vital records are kept in a secure location away from the house (e.g. in a safe deposit box). Consider investing in a safe that is resistant to fire if you intend to keep the items in your own house. In the event that there is water inside the safe, you should be sure to place any important documents in plastic bags.

10) If you have pets, it is in your best interest to prepare contingency arrangements for their care in the case of a natural or man-made disaster. Make sure that you have all of the essential tools and materials for your pet, such as food, water, and an identifying tag, before you bring it home. In addition, it is important to

check that the medical records of your pet are up to date (and that you have a copy of these records, if at all feasible) and that your pet has received all of the necessary immunizations or vaccinations.

Contacting the animal shelter or emergency department in your area might provide you with information that is specific to the region you reside in.

Planning That Is Not Required:

11) Take a First Aid Class: In order to be completely ready for any circumstance in which a disaster may occur, it is always a good idea to take a first aid class. This will allow you to be as prepared as possible.

Making a disaster supply kit

Putting together a disaster supply kit is an efficient approach to ensure that you are organized and well-prepared in the event that a catastrophe befalls your location.

In the event that a catastrophe does take place, you may discover that in order to survive, you will need to do it without the assistance of conveniences that are used on a daily basis, such as electricity or running water. It is of the utmost importance to initiate preemptive preparations for a scenario like this one.

When putting together your emergency supply box, the first thing you should focus on doing is packing the essentials. The following is a list of appropriate goods that should be stowed away in an emergency supplies kit:

1) Food and Water: In the event that you are unable to access food or water from outside sources as a result of the disaster, it is imperative that you be prepared. Make sure that each member of the family has at least three days' worth of food and water stored away in case there is an emergency. It's a good idea to have enough food for at least a fortnight's worth of meals stashed up in case of an emergency, but it really depends on the kind of catastrophe you're preparing for.

   Purchasing commercially bottled water is the most dependable method for storing water in your disaster supply kit, as this will provide a safe form of drinking water in the event of a disaster. If you do not purchase commercially bottled water, you will need to find another way to store your water supply. The current guidelines for water intake stand at around two liters of water per day for every individual. When putting up your emergency supply kit, remember to take this into consideration so that you may stockpile sufficient quantities of water for everyone in the family.

There are a variety of ways water can be stored for use in the event of an emergency; however, purchasing water in commercially packaged bottles is the approach that offers the most level of protection.

It is entirely up to you whether or not you want to make your own water bottles. In the event that this is the case, you should make an effort to obtain suitable containers from a store that specializes in camping supplies and ensure that you clean these well. If you are going to be choosing your own containers, look for bottles that were once used to hold carbonated beverages. Do not use containers that have previously held milk or juice since these products leave behind protein and sugar residue that can encourage the growth of germs that are toxic to humans in your water supplies. Once more, ensure that the containers are completely clean before using them.

After you have acquired your containers and ensured that they are clean, you should next fill them with water and ensure that the lids are securely fastened.

Avoid carrying items that are heavy in salt when you are putting together supplies for the family's meals (as these will make you thirsty and want to drink more). It is imperative that you choose foods that do not need to be refrigerated, such as those that come in cans or are dry. Make sure you have a can opener with you if you intend to bring any food that is tinned.

If there is a member of your family who has certain dietary requirements, you need to make sure that you take this into consideration and provide food that is suited to their needs.

2) Flashlight with extra batteries: Bear in mind that in the event of a disaster, you may be compelled to fend for yourself without the luxuries of normal life, including the use of electricity. Therefore, you should include a flashlight with extra batteries. Be ready for anything by carrying a flashlight or another source of light with you at all times.

3) A television or radio that is powered by a portable battery: You will be able to maintain your awareness of the current situation as well as the procedures that are being carried out if you bring along just one of these objects. Rather than relying on energy, make sure that these items can be powered by batteries.

4) First Aid Bag An emergency supply kit cannot be considered complete without a first aid kit. In the event of a disaster, you may sustain more serious injuries, but you may also find that you are unable to reach a hospital or that hospital services are "backed up." This is in addition to the possibility that you will sustain less severe injuries. Be sure to bring a first aid kit with you so that you can treat any injuries or illnesses that may arise before you can reach a hospital.

5) Sanitary Items: These may contain toilet paper, paper towels, baby wipes, or any other sort of sanitary product you believe may be required.

6) Equipment for the kitchen and cooking: In the event that you are forced to evacuate your home, you will likely need utensils with which you can cook. Bring along the essentials, such a saucepan, a frying pan, and a couple different spoons, for example. Be careful not to go crazy and pack everything except the kitchen sink. Keep in mind that you might be asked to bring your emergency supplies kit with you. It is highly recommended that you bring along a portable cooking equipment of some kind; if you already have one, great! Cooking utensils that are appropriate include candle warmers, fondue sets (for use indoors), and camp stoves (for outdoor use)
Pack a box of matches in an airtight container and include it with the culinary supplies you're bringing. In any given circumstance, these might prove useful.

7) Photocopies of all forms of identification: Put these in your bag in case you end up losing the original documents.

8) Additional garments and blankets The weather in the region in which you live should be taken into account when deciding what kinds of clothes to bring. Bring along enough clothes to see you through several days. In the event that you are required to evacuate, you will be thankful that you did so in advance.

9) Have Some Cash on Hand Be ready for anything, and always have some cash on hand. In the event of a crisis, it is possible that there would be no more access to credit card facilities or automated teller machines (ATMs).

10) Prescriptions Appropriate If you or any member of your family suffers from a medical condition, make sure you pack an adequate supply of necessary medications or medical equipment, as it may not be feasible to obtain these in the event of a disaster. Make it a habit to check the expiration dates of any drugs that are stored in your emergency supplies kit on a frequent basis.

The list that was just presented is a very basic advice that should be followed in order to guarantee that a disaster supplies pack is adequately stocked. Every family is unique and will have its own set of requirements to satisfy. When customizing your emergency supply kit, be sure to take into account the aforementioned factors. It is important to remember to upgrade the kit as your family expands and evolves so that it can continue to meet the needs of the members of the family.

It is imperative that you continue to maintain a disaster supplies kit once you have established one. To get the most out of the life of the dried or canned goods, be sure to keep them stored and sealed in an area that maintains a cold and dry climate for the food. You should make it a habit to perform routine inspections of the contents of your disaster supplies kit and to throw away any canned foods that have dents in them or that have passed their expiration date. It is very advised that all of the food and water be changed out once every half a year.

Be sure to replace any supplies that you use up as you go along.

Managing an evacuation that has occurred

The strategy of evacuating the area is one that is utilized regularly in the event of an emergency. In the event that an evacuation is required, being familiar with the protocols that will be followed and having a game plan prepared in advance will ensure that you are ready for the event, able to keep your cool and maintain control of the situation, and will give you the ability to deal with whatever arises.

You will be informed of the necessity of an evacuation through either the television or the radio, as these are the primary modes of communication. The magnitude of the catastrophe will determine how long you have before you are required to evacuate the location you are at right now. This could be a matter of one or two days in certain circumstances. However, in many instances, evacuating the area may be necessary immediately, which leaves no time to get sufficient supplies. For this reason, being prepared is really necessary.

The items on the following list will be helpful in efficiently managing an evacuation. If there is not enough time, implementing some of the hints might not be possible:

1) If you know you will need to drive in an emergency, make sure the gas tank is always full. In the event of a crisis, gas stations might be forced to close. It is essential, therefore, that you make certain you are well-prepared before the event. If you do not have a car ensure you make arrangments for transportation.

2) Make sure to pay attention to all of the guidance offered by the appropriate authorities.

3) If there is still time, you should definitely put together a disaster supplies kit. Refer to chapter three for instructions on assembling an emergency supplies kit.

4) In the case that an evacuation is ordered, you should get going as soon as you can so that you can avoid becoming stuck in traffic or being held up by the weather.

5) If you are being evacuated from your home and have time to change, make sure that you are wearing shoes that are comfortable and sturdy as well as protective clothing such as long pants.

6) Before you leave your house, take the time to disconnect any electrical appliances, secure any loose items outdoors, and lock the doors and windows.

7) Stay vigilant if you are behind the wheel of a vehicle. Always stay on the main highways and avoid taking any shortcuts. Keep an eye out for any downed electrical wires and keep away from them.

If, for whatever reason, you find yourself in a situation in which you are obliged to leave without sufficient time to plan or pack, the following expedient checklist will assist you in grabbing a few things that may be necessary in the situation. Keep in mind that you should only stop to gather these items if there is sufficient time, and that you should never put your safety in jeopardy in order to do so. If the authorities have demanded that you immediately vacate your place of residence, you are required to comply with their instructions.

1) Don't forget to bring your mobile phone, wallet, and a written list of relevant phone numbers with you. In addition to having these numbers saved in your phone, it is a good idea to jot them down on paper as well. In the unfortunate event that your phone battery dies, you will still have access to them.

2) Assemble some ready-to-eat food and bottled water in a hurry and pack them in your bag.

3) You need to quickly pack a little bag with some extra clothing, some underwear, and some amenities. Make sure you bring along any necessary medications in the appropriate containers.

4) Snag the keys to your house and vehicle and get ready to go.

5) If you have the opportunity, you should bring along a flashlight, a radio that runs on batteries, a supply of spare batteries, and a first aid kit.

In spite of the fact that they can only satisfy the most fundamental requirements, the things in this category will make an evacuation a great deal more tolerable.

Having a prefabricated disaster supplies kit is always important, as this will help ensure that you are not caught off guard during an evacuation and will allow you to avoid being unprepared. Because of this, you will be able to flee the area at the drop of a hat without having to first collect the stuff you need to take with you. Please go to chapter three for information on how to put together a simple emergency supply kit.

Managing an unexpected situation while turning off your utilities

In many different types of situations involving an emergency, the authorities may ask you to turn off the utilities that service your house. Generally speaking, this is done for reasons relating to safety.If you are aware with the procedures involved in turning off the utilities, you will be able to successfully handle the situation in a calm and sensible manner.

The type of emergency that has struck will dictate which services of your home's utilities you are needed to turn off:

1) Turning off the gas supply In the aftermath of a catastrophe, the gas supply is typically turned off to avoid the spread of fire. Depending on their location, states and countries use a variety of unique methods to turn off the power. Get in touch with your gas provider so that you may become familiar with the steps required to turn off the gas supply to your residence.
It is crucial that every member of the family is aware of how to complete this task, so make sure that they all hear the procedure.

   If you find yourself in a situation where you have to shut off the gas, make sure that you have a trained professional restart it.

2) Water: If there is a disaster, there is a chance that a broken pipe in the main water supply could taint the water that is delivered to your home because of a

contaminated main supply. Because of this, there are instances when you have to turn off the water supply that goes to your house.

Find the main house valve that controls the water supply to your home (it may be helpful to know this ahead of time, so that you don't have to waste time looking for it in an emergency situation), and then simply turn the valve so that it is closed. This will effectively cut off the water supply to your house. Check to see that the valve is closed all the way. Once the authorities give the all clear to do so, you will be able to turn the water back on again.

Because water valves have a propensity to rust, you need to make sure that you check yours on a regular basis and replace it if necessary. In the event of an unexpected circumstance, this will make it much simpler to open and close the valve.

3) Electricity: If there is a risk that gas is leaking, you can be asked to turn off your electricity. Sparks from an electrical device have the capability of igniting gas, which can then lead to an explosion.
Find your home's circuit box if you need to turn off the electricity at your residence (it may be useful to know the location of your circuit box ahead of time, this will save time and confusion in the event of a disaster).

Turn off the power to the entire circuit box by first turning off each individual circuit and then turning off the main circuit breaker.

You need to make sure that all of the responsible members of your household know how to turn off the electricity.

Managing during a disaster

Things have the potential to become quite disorderly and unclear when a calamity strikes. The following information is presented to you in the hopes that it will help to clarify any questions or concerns that you may have during this time.

Taking Shelter: Before a tragedy occurred, you should have talked about the importance of designating some rooms as shelters in which people may go to stay safe during the event. The number of rooms available in a shelter will change based on the type of catastrophe.

In the event that you are compelled to leave your house and have not made any other plans for a safe place to stay, public mass shelters are typically available to everyone who needs them. In order to stay in a mass shelter, you will need to cohabit with a significant number of other individuals within a constrained area. Unfortunately, this will not be the most enjoyable experience; but, it will offer you some degree of protection and a roof over your head. Even while food, water, and other necessities for sanitary needs are provided at mass shelters, it is still beneficial for you to have your disaster supplies kit with you in the event of an emergency. This is especially true if a member of your family has specific needs.

In order to maintain proper sanitation, community shelters do not permit the presence of dogs.

Managing Water: In spite of the fact that we see it on television very frequently, it is essential to keep in mind that we should not ration water (unless specified by authorities). Give everyone in the family the opportunity to drink to their satisfaction. If you are prepared and have put together a disaster supplies kit, you ought to have done so taking into account the necessity of having water on hand. The amount of water that a person needs to consume on a daily basis is around two liters. Staying indoors where it's cold and avoiding vigorous activity are two of the best ways to reduce the amount of water you need to drink and, as a result, get the most out of the water you've conserved.

If you have the good fortune to have water packed in bottles, it is imperative that you consume this water in order to avoid the possibility of becoming contaminated.

If you do not have access to water contained in bottles that can be sealed, you can receive water from the following sources instead:

- Ice cubes that have melted

- Water that has been drained from a heater

- Juice that has been extracted from canned or tinned fruit

- Water that has been drained from pipes (ensure you have shut the water off at the main valve before draining from pipes)

Be wary of the water that comes out of the pipes after you've drained them. If the water is hazy or if you have any concerns about drinking it, it is recommended that you treat the water first before consuming it. The following is a list of treatment methods:

1) Bringing to a boil The extremely high temperature that is reached when water is brought to a boil can kill any micro organisms present. The water can be disinfected in a way that is both simple and risk-free by boiling it.
   Bring the water to a boil for one minute, then wait at least one minute before drinking it. The flavor of the water can be significantly improved by moving it back and forth between two containers.

2) Distillation: This process will not only remove microorganisms from the water, but it will also successfully remove any other compounds that may be present. To complete this process, you will need to bring water to a boil and then collect the fumes that are produced.

To distill water, bring it to a boil in a pot that has a lid that matches it and a handle on top of it. You should tie a cup to this handle in such a way that the cup will hang in the correct orientation even when the lid of the pot is inverted. In order to prevent the cup from falling into the boiling water, place the lid on the pit in an inverted position while the water is heating up. Cook at a rolling boil for twenty minutes. When you remove the lid from the pot, you will notice that distilled water has collected in the cup (be careful not to drop the cup).

3) Chlorination: If you are unable to boil the water because you do not have the necessary equipment, you can use this method instead.
The addition of common home bleach will make the chlorinating process go more smoothly. The only kind of bleach that can be used is one that has a sodium hypochlorite concentration of between 5.25 and 6 percent and does not have a scent, is not color safe, or is not blended with another kind of cleaner.

Bleach should be added at a rate of 1/8 of a teaspoon for every 3.7 liters of water. Please let this settle for fifteen minutes before proceeding. The combination should have a faint scent of chlorine; if it does not, the procedure should be repeated. If, after adding the second dose of bleach, the water does not emit a scent of chlorine, you should dispose of it.

When it comes to managing your food supply during a natural disaster, it is essential to keep in mind that the standards for food hygiene and safety will still be in effect. Make sure you wash your hands well before touching or preparing any food.

Make sure that food is stored in containers with lids, and that any food that has been left out at room temperature or that has not been properly sealed should be thrown away. Additionally, make sure that all utensils are kept clean.

Garbage of any kind should be taken outside and discarded in a bag that has been hermetically sealed.

The various catastrophic events that could take place, as well as strategies for responding to them

There is a broad spectrum of potential catastrophes that could take place. Even though calamities can strike in any corner of the world, certain regions are more predisposed to certain kinds of catastrophes than others are. This chapter includes a rundown of some of the more widespread natural disasters that can occur pretty much anywhere, as well as advice on how to respond to them effectively.

Floods are characterized by steadily rising water levels, which are often caused by intense storm activity. It doesn't matter where you are in the world, you could be impacted by flooding at any time. If you have reason to believe that flooding could occur in the area in which you currently reside, it is imperative that you maintain an awareness of the most recent developments in the crisis by keeping abreast of the news on the radio or television.

In the event that you are forced to go outside while a heavy storm is occurring, you should be aware that a flash flood may develop. A flash flood is a type of flood that occurs suddenly and is characterized by massive amounts of water that suddenly appear (i.e. an instant flood with no warning). Move to higher ground as quickly as possible in the event of a flash flood.

In the event that a flood worsens to an unacceptable level, authorities could order you to leave your home.If you have the time, you should try to bring any goods or furniture from outside inside the house, and you should position the indoor furniture so that it is as high as it can possibly be (ideally this would be upstairs in a two story house). Remove all of the plugs from the various pieces of electrical equipment.

If you are traveling through an area that is experiencing flooding, you should avoid walking through any moving water, regardless of how shallow it may seem.

If you are driving, you should avoid driving into or through flooded regions. If you notice that flood levels are beginning to rise around your vehicle, you should exit the vehicle and make your way to higher ground.

Floodwaters continue to rise, posing a grave threat to those who are in the area. Many people have lost their lives because they were carried away by a current and perished as a result of the incident.

If you come across someone who is in jeopardy of being carried away by the current, you should do what you can to save them without putting your own life in jeopardy. Hold out a long rod or stick in an effort to pull them out of the water and assist them.

Should you find yourself in a situation where you have to take a person out of flood waters, the first aid treatment that follows could very well end up saving that person's life.

• Position the individual so that they are lying on their back and apply pressure to their stomach in order to expel any water that may be there. Alternately, the individual may choose to lie on their stomach in order to have pressure given to their back.

• If a person is unresponsive, it is possible that mouth-to-mouth resuscitation will be required.

- Use whatever methods are at your disposal to keep the individual warm, including wrapping them in a blanket or exposing them to your own body heat.

- Notify the appropriate emergency services.

Hurricanes are a very severe type of storm or cyclone that frequently develop in tropical regions. Hurricanes are accompanied by severe storms that are characterized by high wind speeds. These storms frequently lead to the formation of tornadoes and storm surges, which are similar to tidal waves in that they are formed when a dome of water is pushed onto the shore by strong winds. In addition, hurricanes typically cause extensive flooding and heavy damage as a result of the heavy rainfall they produce.

If a storm is currently affecting the area in which you reside, you should make it a priority to tune in to the local radio or television station for the most recent updates.

As a result of the powerful winds that are generated by a hurricane, it is highly recommended that any objects that are not securely fastened that are kept outside be brought inside until the winds die down.

It is possible that a hurricane can grow so severe that the authorities will ask you to leave your home and seek shelter elsewhere. In the event that this is the case, you need to make sure you follow all of the directions.

If you find yourself unable to leave your house for whatever reason, it is imperative that you remain inside the house at all times and keep away from any windows or doors that may be open. Put all of the interior doors in their closed positions, and investigate possible ways to reinforce the exterior door frames. You might be required to take refuge on the ground floor of the house in a small interior room or closet, depending on the force of the hurricane. If you are inside a room, get on your stomach and get as low as you can on the floor. If possible, find a substantial item like a table to crawl beneath for protection.

Thunderstorms: Because thunderstorms are such a typical occurrence, many people tend to forget that they have the potential to be quite hazardous. This is a mistake that can have serious consequences.

Lightning is a byproduct of every thunderstorm, and there is also the risk of tornadoes, high winds, heavy rain, and flooding as a result of these weather events.

If you reside in a region that is prone to thunderstorms, you should avoid venturing outside and instead remain indoors during these times. You should ride out the storm in a car if you are unable to seek shelter in a building of any kind.

If you have advance notice that a storm is on its way, you should try to tie down or bring inside any unsecured things that are located outside until the storm has passed. The production of strong winds can frequently result in the displacement of outside goods, which can then result in harm to the structures that are nearby.

It is best to avoid taking a shower during a storm because the plumbing fittings can carry electricity. Even though the likelihood of lightning striking them is low, you shouldn't put yourself in danger by taking such a chance.

If your home phone includes a cord, you should only use it in an absolute emergency because it could also conduct electricity. The fact that cordless and mobile phones do not conduct electricity makes them completely safe to use.

When lightning strikes a home, the spike in electricity that follows can frequently do significant damage to any electrical items that are still connected in to their sockets. During a storm, it is best practice to remove the plug from any electric equipment so that an incident like this does not occur.

Earthquakes: Earthquakes are characterized by a sequence of vibrations of the ground that can often lead to catastrophic damage to neighboring buildings. Earthquakes can also cause serious injuries to people.

If you find yourself in the middle of an earthquake, here are some things you should do:

If you are inside, take refuge beneath a sturdy piece of furniture or crouche down in a corner and protect your head and face with your arms. If you are outside, seek shelter under an overhanging tree or a sturdy piece of furniture.

Make sure that you keep your distance from any doors or windows, as well as anything else that could potentially fall. Stay indoors until the trembling has completely stopped.

If you are outside and near any buildings or other structures that could collapse, move away from them immediately.

After the tremors have stopped, you should be prepared for the possibility of more vibrations or shockwaves occurring. Even though these additional vibrations are typically not as intense as the first vibrations, they may contribute to further undermine structures that have already been harmed by the earthquake. Make sure you keep a safe distance away from any sites that have been damaged.

Tsunamis are a potential hazard for people who live in coastal areas, as earthquakes can trigger their production (also known as a tidal wave). If there is a possibility that a tsunami will strike, you should move inland as quickly as possible to higher ground.

After the wave from a tsunami has passed, it is still unsafe to enter flooded regions until the local authorities say it is okay to go back.

Fire: Whether this catastrophe occurs on a little scale or on a much larger one, fire is one of the most perilous natural disasters since it spreads so rapidly and poses such a high risk. The heat and smoke that are produced by a fire are also two additional factors that contribute to its lethality.

There are some measures you can take to protect yourself and your family from the dangers of a fire in your own home, such as installing smoke alarms. Among these are the installation of smoke alarms on every level of your home and the routine testing of those alarms to ensure that they are functioning appropriately. It is imperative that smoke alarms are changed out at least once every ten years.

If you live in a multi-story structure, you should take precautions to ensure that your windows and doors are not nailed shut and that there are adequate fire ladders available. These measures will make it easier to evacuate the building in the event of a fire.

In the event that there is a fire in your home, it is essential to have a plan for how to get out of each area in the house in the event that the house catches on fire. Please refer to chapter three if you require any additional information regarding the planning of escape routes.

During the evacuation, keep low to the ground so that you can reduce the amount of smoke and other hazardous chemicals that you breathe in. The fire is the source of these hazards. Check the temperature of the door with the back of your hand by feeling the surface of the door at its highest point before opening any door.

If the door is hot, you should not open it; instead, you should look for an alternate way to leave the building.

Before leaving the room, you should make sure the departure route is free and only open the door if it is not hot. If the door is not hot, you should carefully open it. If there are no obstructions in the way of your exit, proceed to leave the room and lock the door behind you.

If during the course of your evacuation your clothing catches fire, you should immediately descend to the ground in order to put out the flames. Do not run because this will only hasten the process of the fire spreading. It is important that every member of the family is familiar with the stop, drop, and roll procedure.

When treating minor burns or burns that are no more than two to three inches in diameter:

• Bring down the temperature of the burn as quickly as you can by washing it with cold water or applying a cold compress.

• Apply gauze to the burn and cover it.

When treating severe burns or burns of a significant size:

> • Immediately seek the assistance of a medical professional.

> • You should not make any attempts to remove garments or to cool burns by submerging them in water. Instead, apply a cool, wet bandage to the burns and cover them up.

> •If it appears that the person has stopped breathing, you should start performing chest compressions.

www.ingramcontent.com/pod-product-compliance
Lightning Source LLC
LaVergne TN
LVHW010304200726
843506LV00014B/3382